Geranium Essential Oil

Benefits, Properties, Applications, Studies & Recipes

by Ann Sullivan

Published in USA by:

Ann Sullivan
217 N. Seacrest Blvd #9
Boynton Beach
FL 33425

© Copyright 2017

ISBN-13: ISBN-13: 978-1548103965
ISBN-10: 1548103969

Table of Contents

Introduction

What are essential oils, and how might they be used for therapeutic purposes?

Essential oils are ultra-potent oils, extracted from plants and flowers that have been utilized in medicine for centuries. Presently, they're most commonly used to supplement pharmaceutical medication, but they can also be an effective alternative to pharmaceuticals if you don't have access to them. Before you dismiss essential oils to support the body's natural defenses against injuries and illness, look at the historical evidence of the oils' therapeutic competence in practice. Your average age-old medical text will demonstrate that essential oils, herbs, and plenty of other natural ingredients have, for thousands of years, successfully enhanced immune function to meet and defeat any number of ailments and injuries. Though traditional medicine is considered "alternative" now, it was once the gold standard. And, frankly, perhaps it still should be, as these natural age-tested remedies can fortify the body's battlements against everything from simple maladies, like headaches, cuts and bruises, to serious diseases, like cancer.

Essential oils are deemed "essential," because the oils are composed of the "essence" of the plant. The difference between essential oils and other oils – like olive oil or vegetable oil, for instance – is that essential oils have high volatility and reduced fixation, which results in faster evaporation, enabling their popular use in aromatherapy.

Even at high temperatures, olive and vegetable oils don't evaporate.

Essential oils are especially necessary when it comes to a major natural or man-made disaster or some potential viral outbreak. In these types of dire situations, you may not have quick access (or any access at all) to your standard pharmaceutical supply; so, essential oils, along with other alternative medicines, will be your go-to wellness aids in the case of social collapse, viral outbreak or devastating natural disaster. When medical access is null and void, alternatives to our modern-day standard are the only chance we have to keep pathogens at bay.

You probably don't realize that you already use essential oils every day. They're in perfumes, shampoos, soaps, ointments...they're even used in furniture polish. Why are they found in so many aromatic products? Well, basically, because essential oils are super concentrated aromatic liquids, so their scent is remarkably strong. Let's put this into perspective: to steam tea, you use a few leaves of peppermint or juniper; to produce a single ounce of essential oil, five whole *pounds* of peppermint or juniper leaves are required. Some sources claim that to produce twelve pounds of essential oil would necessitate an acre of peppermint, juniper, or any other oil you're looking to produce en masse. Unlike vegetable oil, you don't often find concentrated therapeutic-grade essential oils sold in bulk; instead the oils are often sold in easily carried small, dark bottles, perfect for your GOOD bag (Get Out Of Dodge). Which is exactly what this book is aiming to help you do –

get out of dodge with your most vital of essential oils intact, a good supply of geranium essential oil.

Why geranium, you ask? Well, to get you quickly up to speed on this most essential of oils, below we've provided a condensed synopsis of geranium, after which we'll outline in greater detail the oil's history, properties, and common therapeutic uses, so that you – the consumer – might have a better understanding of the oil's benefits and applications. We've even provided supportive remedies for pure geranium, as well as blended recipes that incorporate the valuable oil. Chapter 3 will further detail past scientific research on geranium essential oil.

Now, let's get down to it.

Essential Oil 101: the Basics of Geranium

Summary: Geranium, or Pelargonium graveolens, has been used for thousands of years as a fragrance, a calming agent, a skin revitalizer, and for therapeutic purposes. In ancient Egypt, geranium was used specifically to brighten and revitalize the skin.

Description: Geranium oil is commonly extracted through steam distillation. The leaves are most often used. The oil is clear or amber in color, thin in consistency, and has a very strong sweet floral scent.

Uses: Beyond those applications previously mentioned, additional uses for geranium essential oil include strengthening the body's defenses against skin conditions, like dull skin, acne, cellulite, oily skin, psoriasis, eczema, and itchiness. It has also been used to support menopause, hepatitis, fungal infections, fatty liver, diabetes, viral conditions, hormone imbalance, digestion, lice, circulatory issues, gallbladder, and menstrual issues, like heavy flow, PMS and cramps. When it comes to mood and emotion, geranium oil calms the nerves and helps to release negative energy.

Properties: Antioxidant, antibacterial, anti-inflammatory, astringent, diuretic, insect repellant, sedative, tonic, hemostatic, cicatrisant, vermifuge and vulnerary properties.

Application: Dilute 1:1 with a carrier oil. You can apply topically, inhale directly, diffuse or use as a dietary supplement.

Safety Precautions: Geranium has been approved by the FDA for internal consumption and so can be used as a dietary supplement. If you have sensitive skin, dilute heavily or avoid. If pregnant, do not use this oil.

Fun facts: The genus of geranium, Pelargonium, is derived from the Greek word for "stork," which is "Palargos," and was so named because a Geranium's fruit looks like the bill of a stork.

Though Europeans have been defending themselves against evil spirits since the 1600s by planting geraniums in their gardens, the first-time geranium leaves were ever distilled was in 1819 by the French chemist, Recluz.

Chapter 1 – Benefits of Geranium Essential Oil

Geranium essential oil offers several therapeutic benefits; but you may be wondering what these benefits are. In this chapter, we'll take a closer look at the history of geranium and its many uses.

Cultivation of Geranium

Originating in South Africa, the Pelargonium genus produces species of evergreen perennials which are highly tolerant of heat and drought, but do not like cold or frosts. In certain temperate regions, some Pelargonium species enjoy popularity as garden plants. However, the Pelargonium graveolens is an uncommon species, known as "rose geranium." The rose geranium is indigenous to Mozambique, Zimbabwe, and South Africa. Zimbabwe and

Mozambique.

Primarily, all Pelargonium species require sunny, warm, and sheltered conditions in which to grow. Rose geraniums are of the "scented leaf group" shrubby evergreen perennials that are easily propagated from cuttings and are commonly grown for their scent. When the leaves of the plant are bruised or touched, a fragrant aroma is emitted. The leaves are from where the essential oil is commonly extracted, which is commercially used in perfumes, potpourri, or even culinary flavorings.

A History of Geranium

The name Pelargonium is derived from the Greek for "stork," which is pelargós. The plant's seed head is similar in appearance to the beak of a stork. The species of geranium often used for essential oils comes from the Pelargonium genus of flowering plants. This genus classification includes around 200 species of various shrubs, perennials, and succulents, which are known both by the name "geranium" and "storksbills" in the US. What's very confusing when it comes to the scientific classification of geraniums is that Geranium is also the botanical genus of a totally separate group of plants. However, this separate group is related to Geraniaceae, the same family as the Pelargonium genus, and produces "hardy geraniums" or "cranesbills." These plants were, at one time, under the helm of the same genus, Geranium, grouped together by Carl Linnaeus, the famous Swede botanist; but in 1789,

Charles L'Héritier separated them into their two present day categories.

The graveolens species has a long history of used in perfumery. The plant is cultivated largely to distill its foliage, from which a rose scent is pungent. However, various cultivators produce "Graveolens" aromas that are like mint, rose, citrus, nutmeg, coconut, and a variety of fruits.

The flowers and leaves of the rose geranium are also used as a flavoring. Teas, sugars, cakes, jellies, jams, salads, sorbets and ice creams are all flavored with rose geranium. Even some pipe tobacco scents utilize the flower to provide a distinct aroma.

Geranium essential oil is a common byproduct of the flower's cultivation, and it is popularly used in massage therapy, aroma therapy, and natural hemorrhoid applications.

Chemical Components

To generate the essential oil from geranium, the leaves must be steam distilled. This results in the oil's key chemical components, which are primarily linalool, limonene, geraniol, citronellol, geranyl butyrate, geranyl acetate, menthone, myrcene, and alpha pinene.

Main Properties of Geranium Essential Oil

Along with the properties previously mentioned in the introduction, geranium oil possesses antioxidant, antibacterial, anti-inflammatory, astringent, diuretic, insect repellant, sedative, tonic, hemostatic, cicatrisant, vermifuge and vulnerary properties. With such a versatile range, geranium is well equipped to fight off any pathogen in the body's path.

Geranium, as mentioned, is composed of linalool, limonene, geraniol, citronellol, geranyl butyrate, geranyl acetate, menthone, myrcene, and alpha pinene. These components are what instill the enormously beneficial properties within geranium essential oil. We'll outline these properties below.

Antioxidant

Anything high in antioxidants – whether fruit, beans, or essential oils – is a powerful advocate for your body. Antioxidants both protect against free radicals and repair their damage. What are free radicals? Free radicals are destructive chemicals that invade your body, produced by substances both inside and out. Some free radicals (or oxidants) form through normal bodily reactions, like inflammation, metabolism and aerobic respiration. Other free radicals form outside the body, but enter it due to exposure. These include harmful pollutants, toxins, smoking, alcohol, X-rays, and UV rays, to name a few. Although our bodies produce their own antioxidants, these often become damaged as we grow older; thus, introducing antioxidants into our bodies allows these nutrients and enzymes to assist in chemical reactions which destroy the oxidants or free radicals. Geranium essential oil is a moderate antioxidant, aiming to detox the body of free radicals that lead to disease.

Antibacterial

Geranium's antibacterial properties make it a powerful protectant against diseases produced by bacteria, such as oral, digestive and urinary tract bacterial infection. What's great is that, unlike some prescription drugs, geranium has no ill effects on bodily wellness or on the healthy natural flora that exists within the stomach and intestines.

Anticonvulsant

As a nervine and sedative, geranium is also an anticonvulsive, which means it helps relieve and reduce convulsive fits, whether epileptic or induced by another form of nervous or psychological condition.

Antidepressant

When it comes to psychological issues, the uplifting scent of geranium combats negative thoughts and, thereby, depression.

Anti-inflammatory

External or internal inflammation can be reduced using geranium essential oil. For instance, if you or your patient has swollen fingers from arthritis or a swollen knee from a sport's injury, oral application of geranium essential oil may decrease irritation or redness, while also soothing the pain that accompanies inflammation.

Antiseptic

The antiseptic and disinfectant properties of geranium essential oil can be reaped topically, applied directly to wounds, or even through burning; the smoke from the oil may help destroy airborne germs. Internal use will help keep the wounds from becoming infections, while external use will support the body's natural function in inhibiting tetanus.

Astringent

For those who do not know what an astringent is, it's a chemical compound that shrinks body tissues, which means it can aid skin issues and irritations, everything from acne to insect bites. The astringent property of geranium essential oil benefits everything from skin to hair to gums to muscles to intestines. As an astringent, geranium is an anti-agent, combating muscle loss through the ability to strengthen. This astringent property also mean that diarrhea can be relieved through use of geranium essential oil, as well as wound and cut bleeding.

Diuretic

If you're looking to lose water weight and reduce blood pressure, geranium essential oil is your agent. The oil stimulates urination, promoting not only the loss of water weight, but the loss of fats, uric acid, sodium, and other body toxins.

Insect Repellant

You don't have to be covered in a sticky bug spray to keep the mosquitoes at bay; geranium essential oil is a match for even the peskiest of bugs. Whether diffused in the bug-infested area or applied topically with a few drops in your favorite skin cream, the strong insecticidal properties will stave off the bugs and will smell great doing it.

Sedative

As a sedative, geranium sedates and calms by reducing anxiety, excitement or irritability. Though sedatives, alone, do not alleviate pain, they do calm the patient, making them less stressed and more compliant.

Tonic

Geranium essential oil benefits each of the body's systems, whether nervous, digestive, respiratory or excretory, making it an unbeatable general tonic. The oil also supports the immune system by helping the body absorb nutrients.

Hemostatic

As a hemostatic agent, geranium essential oil stimulates muscle, skin, gum, hair follicle and blood vessel contraction. In this way, it promotes blood clotting, and so can be used to accelerate the clotting process when a person is bleeding profusely.

Cicatrisant

Applied topically, geranium is effective when it comes to skin issues. The oil fades scars and other skin imperfections, such as acne, boils, stretch marks, and pox. It's also an incredible anti-agent, reducing the appearance of wrinkles and sun spots, tightening skin and providing an even tone. It does this by replacing old skin cells with new ones.

Vermifuge

As a vermifuge, geranium helps rid of parasitic worms and other internal parasites without significantly damaging the host by killing them or stunning them.

Vulnerary

Whether you want to address an ulcer, a cut, or any internal or external wound, geranium essential oil can be diluted with a skin cream and applied to speed up support while also protecting the wound from becoming infected.

Common Therapeutic Uses

Traditionally used as a calming agent and a skin revitalizer, geranium essential oil remains a significant skin support, protecting against several conditions, whether inflammatory, fungal, or bacterial. Geranium essential oil supports overall wellness and organ function, while mentally uplifting and detoxifying the body. Let's take a closer look at the common uses for this oil.

Depression & Anxiety Disorders

Whether it be physical stress or mental stress, geranium's aroma, in conjunction with its therapeutic properties, enable its use in the support of stress disorders, like upset nerves, anxiety, melancholy, and depression. It can help soothe mental fatigue and refresh cognitive function. The oil induces restful sleep, stimulates concentration, and strengthens overall mental wellbeing.

Alzheimer's and Dementia

Geranium essential oil has been shown to have neuroprotective properties. This is due to the oil's ability to inhibit the nitric oxide production and the expression of inflammatory enzymes in the brain, thus reducing the potential for neuroinflammation. In this way, geranium essential oil can be effectively applied to strengthen the body's defenses against neurodegredation when it comes to Alzheimer's, dementia, or other degenerative diseases.

Detoxifying Agent

Geranium essential oil is an effective detoxifying agent. The oil's components eliminate oxidants that enter the body through such environmental inlets as the foods we eat, the products we use, the air we breathe, the water we wash with, and other like factors. Toxins can cause numerous physiological issues, including heart problems, lung or kidney diseases, or even cancer. What geranium does to eliminate free radicals is to draw the toxins out and transfer them into the urinary tract, where they can be safely removed from the body. Thus, through the oil's high antioxidant content and its ability to stimulate urination, geranium helps cleanse and detoxify the body's systems.

Skin Care

Geranium oil supports the body's defenses against acne, wrinkles, scars, dryness, sagging skin, and other skin issues. The oil's properties invigorate dull skin, while cleansing and eliminating excess oil. Whether using geranium essential oil to defy skin aging or to reduce adolescent skin issues, like pimples and acne, the antiseptic, astringent, and anti-inflammatory properties are superb counter-defenders for skin issues. Geranium essential oil also supports cell wellness and the promotes the regeneration of skin cells.

Women's Wellness

Geranium can significantly benefit women at any age, as it helps balance hormones. Female hormones fluctuate, resulting in the fluctuation of bodily function. In some cases, this hormonal imbalance can impact a woman's daily life. Therefore, administering geranium, particularly during periods of menstrual or menopausal influx, can support the body's natural function. If you commonly experience painful or irregular periods or unpleasant menopausal effects, a geranium application can help relieve your menstrual- or menopausal-related condition. The oil can help young women become regular and relieve painful menstrual cramps, while helping aging women combat unpleasant attributes, like hot flashes and mood-swings, all by better maintaining hormonal balance.

Diabetes

Studies have been done on geranium's relationship to blood glucose levels and, thereby, its potential application to diabetic wellness. What these studies have found is that geranium has some of the highest antioxidant and hypoglycemic activity, allowing it to help maintain a steady blood sugar level and reduce the dangerous drops or spikes that those suffering from diabetes experience.

Safety Precautions & Common Applications

Safety

Certain adverse effects may evolve when using pure essential oils. Some essential oils should not be used when pregnant, for example, as they may cause miscarriage. Allergic reactions, too, may occur, especially when applied topically. Always administer an allergy test before committing fully to topical application. When used with other medications, essential oils may react negatively. If you are on any current prescription medications or have a chronic illness, such as high blood pressure, epilepsy or liver disease, then researching the effects of essential oils against your own personal medical history will eliminate any potentially problematic issues.

Geranium has been approved by the FDA for internal consumption and so can be used as a dietary supplement. If pregnant, do not use this oil. If you have sensitive skin, dilute heavily and test before extensive use. Otherwise, dilute 1:1 with a carrier oil. You can apply topically, diffuse or use as a dietary supplement.

Blends

Oftentimes, essential oils are manufactured as blends of several pure oils. For instance, the Protective Blend of certain brands is a mix of cinnamon, clove, rosemary, and eucalyptus. This blend can be used to boost the immune system to help support colds, viruses and flus. The downside to blends is that the more oils added to the mix, the higher the probability your patient may react negatively to the blend if he/she is prone to allergies. There is also the possibility of phototoxicity when working with blends, particularly if they include citrus oils. Be sure to read your labels before administering.

Regardless of these possible effects, essential oils are a viable option for supporting several conditions. Those looking to support or maintain their own personal wellness, or that of their families', should become educated on the uses of essential oils, their natural remedies and the methods of application. Only then can you begin building your kit of essential oils for survival.

Chapter 2 – Recipes for Geranium Essential Oil

In this chapter, we'll offer various recipes for geranium essential oil, both for pure geranium applications and blends. For pure applications, we've provided the appropriate dosage and method of administration to support specific ailments, from airborne bacteria to wrinkles. When it comes to blends, herbalists and aromatherapists often combine geranium essential oil with grapefruit, lime, rose, lavender, jasmine, and bergamot. We'll offer some fantastic blending options in the second half of this chapter.

Pure Applications

Abandonment

Whenever you're feeling abandoned, pour a drop of

geranium essential oil into your hands, rub your palms together, cup them over your nose, and breathe deeply in and out for several minutes. For added support, diffuse throughout the home.

Agitation

Calm anger, nerves, or agitation by diffusing geranium essential oil throughout the home. You can also apply topically, diluting the oil in a 1:1 ratio with a carrier oil and massing into the solar plexus, over the heart, or in a full-body massage.

Airborne Bacteria

To stave off airborne bacteria during cold or flu season, diffuse geranium essential oil throughout the home. You might also disinfect your car by applying a couple drops of geranium essential oil to a cotton ball and sticking it into the air conditioning vent, which will act as its own diffuser.

Autism

Geranium can help provide emotional balance in autistic children, while at the same time, emphasizing the positive end of the strong emotional spectrum. To apply, dilute geranium essential oil in a 1:1 ratio with a carrier oil and apply topically, massaging into the feet and the base of the neck each night.

Bleeding

If you need to stop up bleeding – from shaving nicks, for instance – apply a single drop of geranium essential oil to the affected area.

Bruises

Accelerate the support process when it comes to bruising by diluting 1-2 drops of geranium essential oil in a 1:1 ratio with a carrier oil; then apply topically over the affected area (do not massage).

Calming

Calm anger, stress or nerves diffusing geranium essential oil throughout the home. You can also apply topically, diluting the oil in a 1:1 ratio with a carrier oil and massing into the solar plexus, over the heart, or in a full-body massage. Moreover, you can pour a drop of geranium essential oil into your hands, rub your palms together, cup them over your nose, and breathe deeply in and out for several minutes.

Cancer

Help strengthen the body's natural defenses against cancer by diluting geranium essential oil in a 1:1 ratio with a carrier oil; then apply topically, massaging into the reflex points of the feet or over the affected area. You can also diffuse throughout the home for overall wellness.

Capillaries

For broken capillaries, dilute geranium essential oil in a 1:1 ratio with a carrier oil and apply topically to affected area (do not massage).

Circulation Stimulant

Boost blood circulation by diluting geranium essential oil in a 1:1 ratio with a carrier oil, then apply topically, massaging the application over the heart and into the extremities.

Convulsions

Eliminate convulsions by supporting your body's balance and calming the nervous system. Dilute geranium essential oil in a 1:1 ratio with a carrier oil and massage into the reflex points of the feet, into the back of the neck, and into the affected area three times daily. You can also diffuse throughout the room on a regular basis.

Diabetes

Regulate blood sugar and insulin levels by diluting geranium essential oil in a 1:1 ratio with a carrier oil and applying topically over the pancreas.

Diarrhea

If you're experiencing diarrhea, geranium essential oil is the answer. Apply topically by diluting the oil in a 1:1 ratio with a carrier oil and massaging it into the abdomen in a counterclockwise motion, or place a drop of the oil in your drinking water throughout the day.

Dysmenorrhea

Dysmenorrhea, or painful periods, can be avoided by diluting geranium essential oil in a 1:1 ratio with a carrier oil and applying topically over the lower abdomen, as well as into the ankles and the arches of the feet.

Emotional Balance

Geranium essential oil can help provide emotional balance by diluting in a 1:1 ratio with a carrier oil and applying topically, massaging into the chest and over the heart. You can also administer the oil aromatically by diffusing or inhaling directly from the bottle.

Endometriosis

To combat endometriosis, dilute geranium essential oil in a 1:1 ratio with a carrier oil and massage into the lower abdomen and into the reflex points of the feet three times daily.

Forgiveness

To promote forgiveness, diffuse throughout the home or pour a drop of geranium essential oil into your hands, rub your palms together, cup them over your nose, and breathe deeply in and out for several minutes.

Gallbladder Stones

Support the body's natural defenses against gallbladder stones by diluting geranium essential oil in a 1:1 ratio with a carrier oil; then apply topically, massaging the solution over the affected area and into the reflex points of the feet, up to three times daily.

Grief

To uplift the spirit in a time of grief, diffuse geranium essential oil throughout the home or pour a drop of into your hands, rub your palms together, cup them over your nose, and breathe deeply in and out for several minutes. You can also apply topically, diluting the oil in a 1:1 ratio with a carrier oil and massaging it into the chest, over the heart.

Hair (Dry, Fragile, or Loss)

For damaged, dry or fragile hair or to reduce hair loss, place 15-20 drops of geranium essential oil in a 10-ounce spray bottle of distilled water. Spray on your scalp and let soak before washing as usual. You can also add a drop to your regular individual shampoo application.

Hernia

Hernias can be targeted with geranium essential oil by

diluting in a 1:1 ratio with a carrier oil and applying topically, massaging gently over the affected area twice daily.

Hormone Balance

Regulate hormonal balance by diluting geranium essential oil in a 1:1 ratio with a carrier oil and massaging into the reflex points of the feet or over the pituitary gland. You can also inhale directly from the bottle every day to help maintain balance.

Impetigo

Combat skin irritations like impetigo by diluting geranium essential oil in a 1:1 ratio with a carrier oil and applying topically to the infected area. The oil will relieve the skin and promote support.

Inflammation

Calm inflammation by diluting 1 or 2 drops of geranium essential oil in a 1:1 ratio with a carrier oil, then apply topically, massaging it over the affected area towards the heart and into the reflex points of the feet several times daily.

Insect Repellant

Repel pesky insects by diluting geranium essential oil in a 1:1 ratio with a carrier oil and applying topically to the skin. You can also diffuse throughout the home or place a drop on a cotton ball and set in any problem areas.

Insomnia

With its calming and relaxing scent, geranium essential oil can combat insomnia and ease you into a dreamless sleep. Dilute geranium essential oil in a 1:1 ratio with a carrier oil and massage into the reflex points of the feet, the forehead, and the back of the neck to trigger nervous system response. You might also diffuse or place a couple drops on your pillow or sheets.

Jaundice

Eliminate jaundice by diffusing geranium essential oil throughout the home or through topical application by diluting in a 1:1 ratio with a carrier oil and applying over the affected area.

Jet Lag

Combat jet lag by diluting geranium essential oil in a 1:1 ratio with a carrier oil, then apply topically in a full-body massage, into the forehead and back of the neck, and into the soles of your feet. You can also diffuse throughout the room to refresh your senses after a long journey.

Libido

Geranium has long been used to stimulate the libido. Diffuse regularly or dilute geranium essential oil in a 1:1

ratio with a carrier oil and apply topically to the soles of the feet, the back of the neck, and over the pituitary gland.

Menorrhagia

To relieve menorrhagia, or abnormally long and painful periods, dilute geranium essential oil in a 1:1 ratio with a carrier oil and massage into the lower abdomen and the reflex points of the feet.

Miscarriage

Following a miscarriage (and after seeing your physician), dilute geranium essential oil in a 1:1 ratio with a carrier oil and massage into the lower abdomen and the reflex points of the feet twice daily.

Methicillin-resistant Staphylococcus aureus (MRSA)

MRSA is an infection that results from a strain of staph bacteria which is now resistant to common antibiotics. You can target it with geranium essential oil by diluting in a 1:1 ratio with a carrier oil and massaging over the chest, the soles of the feet, and the affected area. This will simultaneously fight off the infection and stimulate immune response.

Osteoarthritis

To alleviate the inflammation and pain of

osteoarthritis, dilute geranium essential oil in a 1:1 ratio with a carrier oil and massage the solution into the affected area.

Osteoporosis

Similarly, to alleviate the inflammation and pain of osteoporosis, the same application applies; dilute geranium essential oil in a 1:1 ratio with a carrier oil and massage the solution into the affected area.

Pancreas Support

Geranium essential oil promotes pancreas function. Dilute in a 1:1 ratio with a carrier oil and apply topically over the pancreas or massage into the soles of the feet. You might also use it as a dietary supplement.

Paralysis

Ease paralysis through both topical and aromatherapy administration. Diffuse geranium essential oil throughout the home or dilute the oil in a 1:1 ratio with a carrier oil and massage the solution into the affected area, the soles of the feet, and into the spine every day.

Pelvic Pain Syndrome

To relieve the pain of pelvic pain syndrome, dilute geranium essential oil in a 1:1 ratio with a carrier oil and apply topically, massaging into the affected area up to three times daily.

PMS

Alleviate PMS symptoms by diffusing throughout your cycle. You can also dilute geranium essential oil in a 1:1 ratio with a carrier oil and massage it into the reflex points of the feet on a regular basis throughout the month.

Post-Labor

To support post-labor support, dilute geranium essential oil in a 1:1 ratio with a carrier oil and massage into the lower abdomen and the reflex points of the feet several times daily.

Rheumatoid Arthritis

To combat the pain and inflammation of rheumatoid arthritis, dilute geranium essential oil in a 1:1 ratio with a carrier oil and apply topically, massaging the oil into the joints. You can also simply diffuse or steam two drops of the oil in a pan of water. Then remove the steaming pan from the stove, pour into a bowl, place a towel over your head and inhale. If you don't feel it's done its job the first time, you can reheat that same water and use it once more without adding more oil.

Shingles

Relieve and eliminate shingles by diluting geranium essential oil in a 1:1 ratio with a carrier oil; then apply topically, massaging the oil over the affected area. You can also add a few drops to a warm compress and place over the affected area or add a few drops to a warm bath.

Skin (Dry, Sensitive, Eczema, Psoriasis, etc.)

Geranium essential oil can be used for all sorts of skin conditions. Dilute in a 1:1 ratio with a carrier oil and apply to the affected area or substitute a drop or two into your daily skin care regimen.

Stressful Environmental

Combat stress by steaming two drops of geranium essential oil in a pan of water, remove the steaming pan from the stove, pour into a bowl, place a towel over your head and inhale. If you don't feel it's done its job the first time, you can reheat that same water and use it once more without adding more oil. You can also diffuse throughout the room or place a drop onto your shirt collar for portable stress relief. For topical application, dilute geranium essential oil in a 1:1 ratio with a carrier oil and massage into the chest over the heart and into the reflex points of the feet.

Trust

Promote trust by diffusing geranium essential oil throughout the home. You can also apply topically, diluting the oil in a 1:1 ratio with a carrier oil and massing into the solar plexus, over the heart, or in a full-body massage. Moreover, you can pour a drop of geranium essential oil into your hands, rub your palms together, cup them over your nose, and breathe deeply in and out for several minutes.

Ulcer (Gastric)

Target ulcers internally by placing a drop in each meal or glass of water, or externally by diluting geranium essential oil in a 1:1 ratio with a carrier oil and applying topically, massaging into the stomach, the affected area, and into the reflex points of the feet.

Vertigo

Combat vertigo and maintain balance by diffusing geranium essential oil throughout the home. You can also apply topically by diluting in a 1:1 ratio with a carrier oil and massaging into the forehead, the back of the neck, or in a full-body massage. For further support, inhale directly as needed.

Wrinkles

Protect against wrinkles by diluting geranium essential oil in a 1:1 ratio with a carrier oil and massaging over the affected area. You can also add a drop or two to your daily skincare regimen. Be careful around the eyes.

Blends

Acne

Ingredients

- 1 drop Geranium Essential Oil
- 5 drops Melaleuca Essential Oil
- 6 drops Lavender Essential Oil
- 4 ounces Carrier Oil

Directions

To eliminate acne, combine all essential oils in a jar, blending well. Apply topically to the face in place of your daily cleanser, particularly to the affected areas. Use as needed, blending well before each use.

Ankle Swelling Relief

Ingredients

- 3 drops Ginger Essential Oil
- 3 drops Lemon Essential Oil
- 3 drops Geranium Essential Oil
- 3 drops Lavender Essential Oil
- 1 Tbsp. Grapeseed Oil

Directions

To reduce ankle swelling during pregnancy, combine all
ingredients and apply directly to the affected area
several times each day, massaging the feet and ankles
upwards, toward the heart.

Anti-Anxiety Bath

Ingredients

- 2 drops Basil Essential Oil
- 2 drops Grapefruit Essential Oil
- 2 drops Geranium Essential Oil
- 3 drops Lavender Essential Oil
- 3 drops Ylang Ylang Essential Oil

Directions

To wind down, de-stress, and combat anxiety, add all ingredients to your bathwater and stir to disperse. Then inhale deeply while you soak for 20 minutes, but avoid getting water in your eyes, as it may sting.

Brittle or Damaged Hair

Ingredients

- 15 drops Sandalwood Essential Oil
- 10 drops Lavender Essential Oil
- 5 drops Geranium Essential Oil
- 1 ounce Jojoba Oil

Directions

To repair damaged or brittle hair, mix all ingredients in a small container until well combined. Massage into dry hair, place a shower cap over your head, and let sit for 20-30 minutes. Wash hair twice with shampoo to remove excess oil.

Cirrhosis of the Liver

Ingredients

- 2 drops Grapefruit Essential Oil
- 2 drops Clove Essential Oil
- 1 drop Geranium Essential Oil
- 1 drop Rosemary Essential Oil
- 1 tsp Carrier Oil

Directions

To support the liver and combat cirrhosis, combine all ingredients and apply topically over the region of the liver twice daily.

De-stress Massage

Ingredients

- 5 drops Geranium Essential Oil
- 5 drops Coriander Essential Oil
- 5 drops Lavender Essential Oil
- 3 drops Sweet Orange Essential Oil
- 2 ounces Sweet Almond Oil

Directions

To wind down, de-stress, and combat anxiety, combine all ingredients in a small bowl or glass jar and mix well. Apply in a full-body massage.

Earache

Ingredients

- 1 drop Basil Essential Oil
- 1 drop Geranium Essential Oil
- 2 drops Carrier Oil

Directions

To relieve the pain from earaches, combine all ingredients and apply on the ear's surface, as well as behind the ear. You can also add a drop of each oil to a cotton ball to be placed over the ear canal, but do not press inside the ear.

Facial Blend

Ingredients

- 4 drops Neroli Essential Oil
- 2 drops Lavender Essential Oil
- 2 drops Sandalwood Essential Oil
- 1 drop Geranium Essential Oil
- 1 drop Ylang Ylang Essential Oil
- ½ ounce Almond Oil
- ½ ounce Rosehip Oil

Directions

For a fresh facial blend, mix all ingredients in a small jar or container until well combined. Massage in a circular motion into the face, avoiding the eyes. Use as needed as a substitute for your daily moisturizer.

Female Fertility Rub

Ingredients

- 3 drops Ylang Ylang Essential oil
- 5 drops Eucalyptus Essential Oil
- 5 drops Lavender Essential Oil
- 5 drops Cypress Essential Oil
- 10 drops Basil Essential Oil
- 10 drops Frankincense Essential Oil
- 15 drops Geranium Essential Oil
- 15 drops Marjoram Essential Oil
- 25 drops Clary Sage Essential Oil
- 2 Ounces Carrier Oil

Directions

To improve chances of fertility, combine all ingredients in a small bowl, blending well. Massage into the reflex points of the feet two or more times a day. Store in a glass bottle.

Fingernails/Cuticles

Ingredients

- 3 drops Lemon Essential Oil
- 3 drops Geranium Essential Oil
- 3 drops Rosemary Essential Oil
- 6 drops Clary Sage Essential Oil
- 6 drops Lavender Essential Oil
- 1 ounce Jojoba Oil
- 1 ounce Sweet Almond Oil

Directions

To promote healthy nails and cuticles, especially after exposing your hands to harsh chemicals, combine all ingredients in a small bowl, blending well. Before you go to bed, apply a single drop topically to each nail and cuticle, massaging over the nail.

Hemorrhoids

Ingredients

- 5 drops Geranium Essential Oil
- 1 drop Marjoram Essential Oil
- 1 drop Cypress Essential Oil
- 1 drop Lavender Essential Oil
- 1 Tbsp. Carrier Oil

Directions

To relieve hemorrhoids during pregnancy, combine all ingredients in a small bowl, blending well. Apply to the affected area then soak in a sitz bath for 10 minutes.

Hemorrhoids II

Ingredients

- 2 drops Clary Sage Essential Oil
- 2 drops Helichrysum Essential Oil
- 2 drops Geranium Essential Oil
- 2 drops Cypress Essential Oil
- 1 Tbsp. Carrier Oil

Directions

To relieve hemorrhoids during pregnancy, combine all ingredients in a small bowl, blending well. Apply to the affected area then soak in a sitz bath for 10 minutes.

Hot Flash Relief

Ingredients

- 2 drops Peppermint Essential Oil
- 2 drops Clary Sage Essential Oil
- 4 drops Geranium Essential Oil
- 4 drops Bergamot Essential Oil
- 10 drops Lavender Essential Oil
- 8 ounces Witch Hazel (alcohol free)

Directions

To help relieve hot flashes, combine all ingredients in a glass spray bottle and use as needed. Shake vigorously before each use.

Immune Support

Ingredients

- 1 drop Cinnamon Essential Oil
- 2 drops Melaleuca Essential Oil
- 2 drops Eucalyptus Essential Oil
- 2 drops Geranium Essential Oil
- 2 drops Thyme Essential Oil
- 2 ounces Sweet Almond Oil or Body Lotion

Directions

To support the immune system and clear the mind, mix all ingredients in a small bowl or container until well combined. Massage into the reflex points of the feet or use in a full-body massage.

Insect Repellant

Ingredients

- 5 drops Citronella Essential Oil
- 10 drops Geranium Essential Oil
- 10 drops Eucalyptus Essential Oil
- 10 drops Cedarwood Essential Oil
- 10 drops Pennyroyal Essential Oil
- 1 tsp Emulsifier
- 4 ounces Distilled Water

Directions

To blend an effective natural insect repellant, combine essential oils in a spray bottle and shake well. Add the emulsifier, shake again. Finally, add the distilled water and shake. Spray as needed, shaking well before each use.

Jet Lag

Ingredients

- 4 drops Geranium Essential Oil
- 4 drops Peppermint Essential Oil
- 10 drops Rosemary Essential Oil
- 50 mL Carrier Oil

Directions

To enliven your spirits after a long trip, place all ingredients into a small bowl or container and blend thoroughly. Apply topically in a full-body massage.

Alternatively, you can add all ingredients to your bathwater and stir to disperse. Then inhale deeply while you soak for 20 minutes. Avoid getting water in your eyes, as it may sting.

Joyful Blend

Ingredients

- 1 drop Lavender Essential Oil
- 1 drop Clary Sage Essential Oil
- 1 drop Roman Chamomile Essential Oil
- 1 drop Geranium Essential Oil

Directions

To promote joy and euphoria, diffuse this blend throughout your home.

Menopausal Blend

Ingredients

- 1 drop Angelica Essential Oil
- 1 drop Jasmine Essential Oil
- 2 drops Clary Sage Essential Oil
- 5 drops Geranium Essential Oil
- 6 drops Lemon Essential Oil
- 2 ounces Sweet Almond Oil or Body Lotion

Directions

In a small bowl or container, mix all ingredients until well combined. Massage into the reflex points of the feet or add 2 teaspoons to your bathwater.

Mood Stabilizer

Ingredients

- 2 drops Lemon Essential Oil
- 2 drops Geranium Essential Oil

Directions

To stabilize your mood, diffuse the oils and deeply breathe in the vapors.

No Limits Spray

Ingredients

- 12 drops Mandarin Essential Oil
- 6 drops Geranium Essential Oil
- 6 drops Clary Sage Essential Oil
- 3 drops Cinnamon Essential Oil
- 48 mL Distilled Water
- 1 mL Vodka

Directions

For a confidence boosting mist spray that leaves you limitless, combine ingredients in a 50mL glass spray bottle and spray throughout your room, study, or vehicle when needed. Shake well before each use.

Perineal Tearing

Ingredients

- 2 drops Geranium Essential Oil
- 5 drops Clary Sage Essential Oil
- 2 Tbsps. Carrier Oil

Directions

In a small bowl or container, mix all ingredients until well combined. To help relieve perineal tearing, apply hourly to the affected area.

Seasonal Allergy Blend

Ingredients

- 3 drops Eucalyptus Essential Oil
- 3 drops Rosemary Essential Oil
- 4 drops Geranium Essential Oil
- 4 drops Helichrysum Essential Oil
- 8 drops German Chamomile Essential Oil

Directions

To relieve or protect against seasonal allergies, place all
Apply solution to your personal inhaler. Use as needed.

Tired Feet

Ingredients

- 1 drop Peppermint Essential Oil
- 2 drops Geranium Essential Oil
- 2 drops Lavender Essential Oil
- 1 Tbsp. Carrier Oil

Directions

To relieve feet, wear and tear, place all ingredients in a bowl or jar and mix thoroughly to combine. Apply solution topically, massaging into the feet.

A second application is to add all ingredients to a warm foot bath. Soak the feet in the solution for 10-15 minutes.

Chapter 3 – Geranium Essential Oil Studies

Many studies have been done on essential oils to uncover and prove their therapeutic qualities. In the case of the great number of geranium studies, many of the properties attributed to the essential oil (noted in this book and elsewhere) are quite often validated through the research from accredited universities and published by reputable scientific journals. In this chapter, we'll discuss a small portion of these studies. It's important to note that our knowledge of essential oils is constantly evolving. Keep up with any recent research, as it may turn up even further valuable uses for these miracle oils.

Study 1 – Antioxidant & Hypoglycemic Activity

In this study published by the *Lipids in Health and Disease*, the antioxidant and hypoglycemic activities of geranium essential oil were examined, with the following results: "Rose-scented geranium (Pelargonium graveolens L'Hér.), which is used in traditional Tunisian folk medicine for the treatment of hyperglycaemia, is widely known as one of the medicinal herbs with the highest antioxidant activity. The present paper is conducted to test the hypoglycemic and antioxidative activities of the leaf essential oil of P. graveolens... [The results] suggest that administration of essential oil of P. graveolens may be helpful in the prevention of diabetic complications associated with oxidative stress. Our results, therefore, suggest that the rose-scented geranium could be used as a safe alternative antihyperglycemic drug for diabetic patients."

In this comparative study, geranium essential oil was tested against the anti-diabetic drug, glibenclamide. The oil was orally administered on diabetic rats for thirty days in two different doses – 75 mg/kg body weight and 150 mg/kg – and the results were evaluated, including the antioxidant components, and the serum glucose and hepatic glycogen levels. The results found that geranium essential oil, especially at the 150 mg/kg dosage, was significantly more effective than the anti-diabetic drug. The serum glucose levels declined significantly, while the antioxidant and hypoglycemic effects of the oil were an improvement upon the control drug. These results indicate the efficacy of using geranium essential oil to support diabetic health as an antihyperglycemic agent.

Reference

http://www.ncbi.nlm.nih.gov/pubmed/22734822

http://www.ncbi.nlm.nih.gov/pmc/articles/PMC3439344/

Study 2 – Antibacterial Properties

In this study published by *Molecules*, the antibacterial properties of geranium essential oil were examined, with the following results: "Acinetobacter sp. represent an important cause of nosocomial infections. Their resistance to some antibiotics, their ability to survive on inanimate surfaces in the hospital environment and their ability to produce biofilms contributes to their virulence. The aim of the study was to determine the antibacterial properties of cinnamon, lavender and geranium essential oils against bacteria of the genus Acinetobacter isolated from several clinical materials and from the hospital environment… The MIC values for geranium oil were between 7.5 and 9.5 µL/mL, and between 10.5 and 13.0 µL/mL for lavender oil. These essential oils can be best employed in the fight against infections caused by bacteria from Acinetobacter genus as components of formulations for hygiene and disinfection of hospital environment."

Acinetobacter baumannii is a Gram-negative bacterium, which can become an opportunistic pathogen, especially in hospital environments, infecting those with compromised immune systems. A. baumannii is highly antibiotic-resistant, putting it in the category of an ESKAPE pathogen (ESKAPE includes the following bacteria: Enterococcus faecalis, Staphylococcus aureus, Klebsiella pneumoniae, Acinetobacter baumannii, Pseudomonas aeruginosa, and Enterobacter species). Being that this bacterium seems to have risen to prominence during the Iraq War in military facilities, A. baumannii is colloquially called the 'Iraqibacter'. The bacteria are particularly relevant to those soldiers and veterans who serve in Afghanistan and Iraq, but a multidrug-resistant strain of the bacteria has found its way into civilian hospitals, partially due to the transfer of infected soldiers to these facilities.

In this study, lavender, cinnamon, and geranium essential oils were tested against clinical strains of this bacteria. Cinnamon bark showed the highest inhibition at the lowest concentration, with geranium and lavender following closely behind. The study indicates that all three of the essential oils demonstrate potential against this strain of bacteria and may be used in the hospital or clinic to disinfect and promote hygiene.

Reference

http://www.ncbi.nlm.nih.gov/pubmed/25514231

http://www.mdpi.com/1420-3049/19/12/20929]

Study 3 – Antifungal Properties

In this study published by *ABP ACTA Biochimica Polonica*, the antifungal effects of geranium essential oil were examined, with the following results: "The influence of essential oils (EOs) used at sub lethal level, on the presence and intensity of Candida albicans virulence factors was evaluated. Minimal inhibitory concentrations (MICs) of Lemon balm, Citronella, Geranium and Clove oils were established as 0.097% (v/v)…Thus, it has been shown that tested oils, used even at subMIC, exhibit significant activity reducing the presence/quantity of important C. albicans virulence factors."

Candida albicans develops as yeast and filamentous cells, and can potentially cause genital and oral infections. C. albicans also increases the probability of mortality in immunocompromised individuals (cancer or AIDS patients, for instance).

This study tested the antifungal effects of several essential oils, including geranium, on two strains of Candida albicans – C. albicans ATCC 10231 and C. albicans ATCC 90028. The results showed that the essential oils significantly reduced the fungi's ability to form germ tubes or penetrate the agar. The oils also debilitated the fungi's adhesion to the fibroblast monolayer, cells of connective tissue found in the human body. These results indicate that the essential oils tested can inhibit the candida strains by reducing their number and their viability.

Reference

http://www.ncbi.nlm.nih.gov/pubmed/24644554]

http://www.actabp.pl/pdf/1_2014/115.pdf]

Study 4 – Antioxidant Properties & Sperm Mobility

In this study published in the *Lipids in Health and Disease*, the antioxidant properties of geranium essential oil were examined, with the following results: "Exposure to the pyrethroid pesticide deltamethrin has been demonstrated to exert a wide range of effects on non-targeted organisms. The beneficial effects of geranium essential oil (EO) as an antioxidant has been assessed in deltamethrin (DL) orally administered mice by studying whether the reprotoxicity caused by deltamethrin can be effectively combated with the geranium oil and the effects were compared to vitamin E, as the standard reference drug…Essential oil of geranium prevented testicular oxidative damage explored by reduced LPP and improved total sperm motility, viability and morphology in mice spermatozoa. Our study showed a positive influence of geranium essential oil in the animal male reproductive system similar than that of Vit E."

This study was a comparative analysis between geranium essential oil and vitamin E when it comes to testicular oxidative damage resulting from the pesticide, deltamethrin, one of the most widely used insecticides globally and commonly used in the US to eliminate fleas, ticks, spiders, ants, cockroaches, bees, and bed bugs. Though considered a "safe" class of pesticides, deltamethrin can cause facial paraesthesia upon contact with the skin, tainted breast milk, and reprotoxicity (toxicity to the reproductive process) in humans.

The objective of this study was to see if geranium essential oil's antioxidant properties might have preventative effects in reprotoxicity. The study found that, when applied to rats with testicular oxidative damage, geranium essential oil had similar efficacy in relation to vitamin E, with improvement in sperm viability, motility, and morphology, accompanied by reduced LPP. This indicates that geranium essential oil may be used as a potential reproductive or fertility support when it comes to testicular oxidative damage.

Reference
http://www.ncbi.nlm.nih.gov/pubmed/23496944]

http://www.ncbi.nlm.nih.gov/pmc/articles/PMC3641007/pdf/1476-511X-12-30.pdf]

Study 5 – Anti-inflammatory Properties

In this study published in *Coaction*, the anti-inflammatory effects of geranium essential oil were examined, with the following results: "Since the available anti-inflammatory drugs exert an extensive variety of side effects, the search for new anti-inflammatory agents has been a priority of pharmaceutical industries. The aim of the present study was to assess the anti-inflammatory activities of the essential oil of rose geranium (RGEO)...Our results indicate that RGEO may have significant potential for the development of novel anti-inflammatory drugs with improved safety profile."

The anti-inflammatory property of geranium essential oil was examined through a test that induced paw edema (fluid swelling in the skin or body cavities) using carrageenan. Three doses of geranium essential oil were administered orally to five different groups of test subjects. The 100 mg/kg dosage significantly reduced the paw edema at a similar degree as the control. Moreover, the oil demonstrated potent anti-inflammatory activity when it came to relieving ear edema through topical treatment. Inflammation was reduced by 88% with a 10 μl dose. These results suggest the potential for geranium essential oil in alleviating issues of inflammation.

Reference http://www.ncbi.nlm.nih.gov/pubmed/24103319]

http://www.ncbi.nlm.nih.gov/pmc/articles/PMC3793238/pdf/LJM-8-22520.pdf]

Study 6 – Antifungal & Anti-inflammatory Activities

In this study published by the *Dentist Research Journal*, the antifungal and anti-inflammatory activities of geranium essential oil were examined, with the following results: "Natural products are proved to play a good role as an alternative to synthetic chemicals in clinical conditions. Previous studies showed that Pelargonium graveolens has anti-inflammatory and antifungal activity against Candida albicans. The aim of this study was to evaluate the efficacy of essential oil of Pelargonium graveolens in the treatment of denture stomatitis...It seems that the application of a 1% Geranium oil topical gel formulation is more effective than placebo in the treatment of denture stomatitis."

This study evaluates the antifungal and anti-inflammatory activities of geranium essential oil regarding denture stomatitis. Denture stomatitis is also known as "denture sore mouth" and "Candida-associated denture induced stomatitis." The condition includes redness and inflammation of the mucous membrane of the mouth beneath dentures. Candida species are responsible for around 90% of the cases of denture stomatitis, which is the most common form of oral yeast infection and is often an issue for elderly folk who wear dentures.

The study divided 80 subjects into two groups of 40 patients each, the control group being treated with a placebo and the experimental group with geranium essential oil in a 1% gel. The subjects applied the gel twice a day over the course of two weeks. The results showed that 34% of the denture stomatitis in the experimental group had improved completely, while 56% had improved partially, and only 10% not at all. This is compared with 5% full improvement, 25% partial, and 70% none in the control group. Fungal growth was significantly reduced through the application of the geranium essential oil gel.

These results indicate that geranium essential oil's anti-inflammatory and antifungal properties can be potentially beneficial to supporting the body's natural defenses against denture stomatitis.

Reference

http://www.ncbi.nlm.nih.gov/pubmed/23372587

http://www.ncbi.nlm.nih.gov/pmc/articles/PMC3556280/?report=reader]

Study 7 – Alzheimer's Disease

In this study published by the *Journal of Functional Foods*, the anti-neuroinflammatory activities of geranium essential oil were examined, with the following results: "Microglial cells are major immune cells in the brain, and their activation is involved in neurodegenerative diseases such as Alzheimer's disease…When tested…at higher concentrations, citronellol exhibited an inhibitory activity. The results suggest a possible synergistic interaction between these components. Thus, geranium oil might be beneficial in the prevention/treatment of neurodegenerative diseases where neuroinflammation is part of the pathophysiology."

Alzheimer's disease involves the development of abnormal clumps of fiber bundles in the brain. These neurofibrillary tangles distribute activated microglia, which over-express IL-1, contributing to the amyloid deposits in Alzheimer's patients' brains. Microglia is also partially responsible for the neuroinflammation and for the secretion of cytokines that are neurotoxic. This progressive, neurodegenerative disease is devastating and results in loss of speech, motivation, and short-term memory, mood swings, and behavioral issues. The disease accounts for 60% to 70% of dementia cases.

The study showed that geranium essential oil inhibited the nitric oxide production and the expression of inflammatory enzymes, thus reducing the potential for neuroinflammation. In this way, geranium essential oil can be effectively applied to strengthen the body's defenses against neurodegredation.

Reference

http://www.sciencedirect.com/science/article/pii/S1756464609000796

Chapter 4 – The Ins & Outs of Essential Oils

Where do essential oils come from?

Plants and plant species naturally produce essential oils for various reasons, one being to draw pollinator insects to them, another being to repel invading organisms (bacteria, animals). Several chemical compounds compose each plant's essential oil, and the combination of these compounds are specific to each oil, which then instills in the oil its own unique properties. Essential oils can be harnessed from all sorts of plant components, including flowers, leaves, bark, fruit, roots, and resin. For instance, cinnamon oil is harnessed from bark, lemon oil from the peel, and lavender oil from lavender flowers. Certain plants can produce a few chemical variants of the same essential oil, which are acquired from different parts of the plant.

Some of these parts produce a large amount of oil, while others produce just a smidgen. The oil's quality and potency depends upon several factors, including the subspecies of the plant, its soil conditions, the time of year and even the time of day you harvest it.

How are essential oils extracted?

Essential oils can be extracted from plants through various methods, including pressing, distillation, solvent and maceration. Let's take a brief look at each:

Pressing Method

Commonly used with citrus fruit, the pressing method extracts the oil through a technique which involves pushing the fruit peels through a press. Oily fruits and plants are best suited for this technique. Orange oil, for example, is extracted from orange skins through the pressing method.

Distillation Method

This technique harkens back to the days of old-timey moonshiners, as the same sort of method used to create strong liquor can be used to extract essential oils. Using a still, boiled water and plant materials will create steam which is then cooled by coils and condensed into a combination of water and oil. This combination doesn't mix, so the oil can then be extracted from it.

Solvent Method

Through a multi-step process, certain plant and flower oils can be extracted using alcohol and other solvents, which extort the essential oil from the plant materials.

Maceration Method

When a "carrier" or fixed oil or lard is mixed with the plant material and set out in the sun, over a period, the carrier oil is infused with the plant's essence. Heat sources, other than the sun, are often used to speed the process. Throughout the process, more plant material is added to produce a more potent oil.

How do you use essential oils?

Although some studies about the effectiveness of essential oils are conducted by small companies or even individuals, several them are conducted by the food and cosmetic industries. In general, the pharmaceutical industry shows next to no interest in herbal medicine, primarily because there are few options to patent such products. Being as such, the product's lack of profitability results in a lack of research funding. Regardless, the historical uses of essential oils tell us what we need to know: these oils have been effectively administered for centuries. The therapeutic qualifications of essential oils can be plotted in the survival of humans across cultures and generations.

Another reason that studies on essential oils have not resulted in much conclusive evidence as to their overall effectiveness is because definitive results are sometimes difficult to prove, as the quality of each batch of oil can vary for several reasons. One is that essential oils are impossible to standardize. As mentioned above, even the slightest variance in soil conditions and the time of harvesting – as well as innumerable other factors – will produce a different product quality and potency. In addition, essential oils are often obtained from various species of the same plant; Eucalyptus radiata and Eucalyptus globulus can both be used in the making of therapeutic-grade eucalyptus oil and, as a result, they may have slightly different properties and degrees of strength or effectiveness.

Just as there are several methods by which to extract essential oils, there are several methods to administer them therapeutically. The variety of chemical compounds in each essential oil means that their benefits and applications also vary across the board. Below are a few of these methods.

Topical Administration

Direct application of many essential oils works like a sponge, as skin sops up chemicals and other things (like sunlight, for instance). Topical application is best when you want to clear up an ailment on the skin's surface or in the underlying muscle tissue. When applying topically, you may either massage the oil into the skin or simply dab on the skin for therapeutic results. You might combine the essential oil with a carrier oil for topical use to dilute its potency. This is safer, as the oil is so concentrated. You may support your body's defenses against rash or muscle pain in this manner, but you should always test your patient for allergens before applying. Adverse effects are produced by natural chemicals as much as synthetic ones; poison ivy, for example.

To test for allergens, place a drop or two on your patient's inner forearm. If a rash develops within 12 to 24 hours, then the patient is allergic. In addition, phototoxicity – sun exposure resulting in an exacerbated burn – may be an issue when citrus oils are applied topically. So, one must proceed with caution when applying essential oils using this method.

Inhalation Therapy

Commonly known as "aromatherapy", this essential oil application is effective for inner ailments, like sore throat or cold. In a steaming bowl of distilled or sterilized water, add a few drops of essential oil and, with a towel over your head, bend over the bowl and inhale. The towel captures the vapors, making the technique even more effective. Essential oils can also be placed in a diffuser or potpourri throughout a room to produce somewhat diluted therapeutic effects.

Ingestion

When using this method, proceed with caution. Direct ingestion of essential oils must be monitored and applied in small doses that are diluted in a tablespoon or more of any carrier oil – olive oil, for example. If you are unsure of dosage amounts, make a tea with the relevant herb instead. Although the effects of this diluted use may be weaker, this application is a better alternative than an overdose of essential oils.

What are the general benefits of using essential oils?

Replacement for Prescription Drugs

One practical benefit for using essential oils is, of course, their substitutive nature. Many believe that they can replace Rx drugs, which is the ultimate reason to educate yourself on their application and to begin stockpiling your essential oil supply. Although it is our opinion that 100% pure essential oils that carry no harmful side effects are better to support the body and its functions, we recommend that you consult your physician before replacing your prescription or over-the-counter medications.

One of the potential threats of economic or social collapse is the lack of resources, and primarily the inability to procure prescription drugs. Being as such, finding suitable alternatives should be a priority when prepping for the worst.

Their portability is also a major bonus when it comes to survival prepping. The fact that these ultra-concentrated oils take up little-to-no space makes toting them to your shelter all the simpler should the need arise. And, because essential oils are highly concentrated, the application used in most procedures requires only a drop or two of oil, which means that tiny bottle will be long-lasting (example 15mL bottle contains approx. 250 drops).

Cheap, but Effective Alternative

Though money may be the last thing on your mind when it comes to prepping for a survival situation (money may even be obsolete in the event of social collapse), it is worth noting that the expense of essential oils pales in comparison to prescription drugs. In fact, whether you are forced to survive on essential oils due to a lack of prescription reserves, in some cases, you might consider substituting your prescriptions for these inexpensive alternatives regardless. Essential oils are a cheap, but equally effective alternative to prescription medicine.

No Expiration Date

Another benefit of essential oils is that they do not expire, neither do they have "proper storage" requirements. Several medicines and therapeutic products must be replaced every couple years, so this sets essential oils ahead of the pack when it comes to shelf life.

Versatility

Essential oils also offer great versatility. Apart from providing wellness benefits, essential oils can be repurposed for household and hygienic applications. For instance, if you're looking for something that might serve your dental hygiene needs in a time of crisis, thieves oil is your go-to essential oil. If you want to maintain your skin's wellness, frankincense and lavender will do the trick; the latter also serves as sunscreen, so you can prevent sun damage as well.

When it comes to the house or shelter, you can use essential oils to deodorize, which will come in handy in a disaster scenario where things might start to smell fishy due to lack of proper utilities and care. For example, after the 2011 tsunami and the subsequent nuclear reactor meltdown in Japan, a nurse named Risa Nakahira used essential oils to deodorize and sanitize putrid public bathrooms in overpopulated evacuation facilities. As relief workers searched for survivors, often wading through debris and decay, Nakahira also deodorized their boots and masks using essential oils. The possibilities of these natural oils are endless.

They are also versatile when it comes to the range of patients they're capable of supporting. The wellness of everyone from your great grandfather to your infant baby can be fortified with the aid of essential oils in the appropriate dosage. They even come in handy when supporting livestock or pets. From teething infants to dementia in the elderly, from teenagers with acne to dogs with urinary tract infections, essential oils can serve any patient with nearly any ailment.

Conclusion

Now that you know all about what geranium essential oil can do for you – where it originates, how it's extracted, its benefits and properties, and the different methods of administration – you can use it confidently to support the body's defenses against wellness issues and start to assemble a kit of essential oils for survival.

The various benefits of essential oils and their properties are countless. To build your own kit, first focus on acquiring the essential oils which may bear more relevance to your wellness issues or the potential wellness threats within your environment. When it comes to skin issues, for instance, geranium essential oil will be one of your more crucial oils, due to its skin rejuvenating properties.

Used as a supplement or as your go-to for women's wellness, detoxification, or anxiety disorders, the application of geranium essential oil in medicine has survived for centuries and will survive centuries more. When it comes down to it, you don't need to rely on pharmaceuticals; essential oils, herbs, and plenty of other natural ingredients can be used to help support any number of wellness issues, whether ailment or injury.

Essential oils are essential to your survival in the case of viral outbreak, social collapse or natural disaster because, when the SHTF, your access to pharmaceuticals will likely either be limited or eliminated altogether. Alternatives to our modern-day standard will equate survival when no other option exists. And when it comes to a life-or-death situation, you can't let your wellness decline, no matter the state of the world.

DISCLAIMER AND/OR LEGAL NOTICES: Every effort has been made to accurately represent this book and it's potential. Results vary with every individual, and your results may or may not be different from those depicted. No promises, guarantees or warranties, whether stated or implied, have been made that you will produce any specific result from this book. Your efforts are individual and unique, and may vary from those shown. Your success depends on your efforts, background and motivation.

The material in this publication is provided for educational and informational purposes only and is not intended as medical advice. The information contained in this book should not be used to diagnose or treat any illness, metabolic disorder, disease or health problem. Always consult your physician or healthcare provider before beginning any nutrition or exercise program. Use of the programs, advice, and information contained in this book is at the sole choice and risk of the reader.